Goodbye Daddy

SPEAK UP BEFORE IT'S TOO LATE

Goodbye Daddy

SPEAK UP BEFORE IT'S TOO LATE

A Social Worker's Journey with
Hospice and Palliative Care

Beverly Dotson

MISSION POSSIBLE PRESS
Creating Legacies through Absolute Good Works

The Mission is Possible.
May you thrive and be good in all you are and all you do…
Be Cause U.R. Absolute Good!

♡
**MISSION
POSSIBLE
PRESS**

© 2017 by Beverly Dotson
All rights reserved.

Books may be purchased in quantity by contacting the publisher directly:
MISSION POSSIBLE PRESS,
A division of Absolute Good,
PO Box 8039 St. Louis, MO 63156
or by calling 240.644.2500.

ISBN: 978-0-9861818-5-6
First Edition   Printed in the United States

James Oliver Dotson, Sr., you always told me that whatever I put my mind and heart to, can be done. Thank you, daddy, for being my rock in life and memory.

Contents

My Daddy

— ❦ —

My father's struggle and ultimate death from kidney failure inspired me to go into the medical profession to support, inform and prepare families. I didn't want anyone else to have the experience we did, and I committed to doing something about it.

My eyes have seen so much that for a time, I had been walking around with a closed heart to shield me from the pain. It started when my dad died. I told myself I didn't want another family to experience what we had. I decided to go into social work to support families in getting the support, answers and hopefully, understanding, they need to make informed choices for their loved ones and themselves.

We had a special relationship. We were so close, and I was a daddy's girl, that made it special. At the point where he was hospitalized, we had no idea that he was dying. Just like so many of our fathers who have hypertension and high blood pressure which lead him to kidney failure – a too often, lethal combination.

When my dad was in the hospital, no one sat down to tell us he was going to die soon. He was a sick man. The doctors were speaking but my mom, with her grade school education, (not taking anything away from her, just speaking the truth) didn't understand what was going on. She just knew my daddy was sick. My brothers and I were just kids when he was diagnosed. James was in high school and Chris and I were in grade school. We just knew he had to go back and forth to the dialysis unit Mondays, Wednesdays and Fridays. Dialysis became his routine. He was wiped out after the treatments and spent days recovering in bed. Dialysis, bed. Bed rest, dialysis. It was his life until his death.

He said what he wanted to say and would care less how you took it. Ornery and stubborn. He was direct, honest and rarely smiled. His stature alone was intimidating. People thought he was a mean man, and they were right. You could not mess with his family. "Old Jabo" is what they called my daddy. He was real protective of us all, and especially me, his only daughter.

It was kind of unexpected that he died. He died on my mom's birthday. He had been ill for so long; I guess we had just gotten accustomed to his dialysis routine and expected that though he was going to treatments, he would remain with us. After all, he had a transplant once. His body rejected it. When I was a teenager, I would sleep in the bed with the phone. You know, after late night phone calls with one of my little boyfriends of the time, most nights I was too tired to put the phone on its base. One afternoon we heard from the hospital that they had tried to call him in the middle of the night to tell him there was a kidney for him and to come in immediately. Unfortunately, they said the phone rang busy after repeatedly calling, so he missed the organ and someone else got it.

They blamed me for my father having missed "his" new kidney because apparently, I left the phone off the hook. He never got another kidney call, as his condition had worsened so much, he wasn't considered a candidate. The pain of thinking I was the cause for missing the kidney has stuck with me for a very long time.

I believe that's when I developed a nervous condition. In high school, I was so self-conscious of everything I did. I would break out with pustules, which looked like hives, on my hands. I would just focus on what was ahead and be a nervous, worried, straight-A student, with an anger problem. I was angry that I had let this happen. I was angry that he was sick. I was angry there was nothing I could do for my daddy.

My grades started going down as he began weeks-at-a-time stays in the hospital. I got angrier; he got sicker. Life got more complex. He ended up living his mean and ornery life for many years, sick and back and forth to dialysis. It wasn't a great quality of life, but he was still with us. It seems that when people are truly mean and ornery, and live their lives like that, they stay around for a long time – bitter, angry, in pain, not-withstanding.

The great thing about my daddy? He never complained. No matter how bad he was hurting, he never complained, that I can recall. He didn't complain until his last day when he said, "My stomach is hurting." Perhaps partly because of his silence and acceptance of the pain, we were blindsided by his death, in a seemingly sudden manner, though he had been on dialysis for 12 1/2 years.

The day he died he had asked me to bring a white shirt, some clean white socks, and clean white underwear to the hospital. When he said that, I asked him where he was going. He didn't answer. Little did I know he was trying to give me a clue that he was getting ready to leave. By this time I was in the health care field, yet I didn't see that one coming. I made sure he had what he requested.

He was looking a bit more tired than his normal, and we decided to let him get some rest. Before I left I asked him if he knew what day it was and he said, "Yes, it's Popeye's birthday." That was my mom's nickname and though they hadn't had a meaningful conversation in a year, my mom was sitting in the corner watching. It's strange to think they hadn't talked but it's just the plain truth – they had a tension-filled relationship as my mother is a nagger, and it grated on him. His response? My daddy used to say little hurtful things to my mom, from insults to curse words. At first, she excused his behavior partly because of his illness (I think he felt less-than-a-man), but mostly because of his mean-spiritedness, then she just stopped talking to him. I felt him saying he was sorry to my mom, without words, the sentiment was in his eyes and body language, that communication they had established through 32 years of marriage.

Remember, I told you he was mean? He didn't even tell her "Happy Birthday," he just acknowledged to me that it was her birthday. Before we left the room, I held my daughter, who was five years old at the time, next to him as he gave her a big kiss and told her he loved her. Mom didn't have much to say other than a quick bye, and I said, "I love you, daddy." He said, "I love you too."

Less than two hours later, we were back at the hospital after receiving the call that he wasn't doing well. My dad had checked into the hospital on a Thursday. He died on Saturday, with a tube sticking out of his mouth because they tried to resuscitate him. The sad part? We had never had an advanced care/directive care conversation nor documents in place. For all those years, no one advised us to get things to make it easier for the loved ones who are transitioning and for those who are left to put together the pieces.

That day I promised God I would do everything I needed to get the education I could, to talk to families.

I've Been Through A Lot

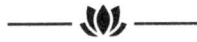

— ❀ —

I've worked in healthcare since the age of 16. I've seen the rudeness of the young and the old, displaying hate toward each other. I've had feces thrown in my face. I have been escorted out of a nursing home by police for advocating for a patient and their family. And I've been assaulted by irate family members during their extreme moments of grief. Believe it or not, I wouldn't change a thing.

As you read my book, you will feel what I've been carrying around for the last 20 years, the demarcation point when my father passed, because it's time to tell it. Too many people don't *Speak Up Before It's Too Late*. That needs to stop. When we open up, everyone benefits.

During my career, I've witnessed the process of families expressing heartaches, disappointments, grief, denial, guilt and pain. I've also witnessed gatherings of relief, respect, admiration and legacies as loved ones say goodbye. During the writing process, I have found healing and understanding in my silent cries. No one knows someone's pain until they share it; whether done verbally, physically or acting out with warm tears sliding down your cheeks. To me, the tears open the door to exploring the "why" inside, giving the strength to ask the necessary questions and take responsible action in the face of trauma and loss. I've seen so much through my own eyes and even more through the eyes of others even in silence, the eyes say it all, be it sadness, happiness, or finality.

I've contemplated writing this book about the experiences and challenges of families I've touched directly or indirectly throughout the years. I think about the countless, sleepless nights when I didn't agree with the decisions of authorities or medical professionals regarding patient care. So many nights I have battled my own countertransferences, putting myself in their shoes, and even the time when a patient looked like my own father, incarnate. None of it has been easy, yet at no time did I believe I could give up. Patients and families need me, just as much as I need them.

Withnessing

— 🪷 —

"We speak with our eyes."

From the moment you simply look at a person, to witnessing a blink or two, or engage in a fixated stare, your eyes are speaking. Have you ever noticed a person's pupils, the glaring reflection in the eyeballs which blink with the slightest contact, the eyelids flicker in a rhythm of their own? What are they saying?

Can you imagine?

You're lying on your back with a breathing tube down your throat hooked up to a ventilator, pumping air into your body. A feeding tube is in your nose giving you liquid nourishment with plastic tubes in the orifices of your body, one in your rectum, and one in your vagina or penis catching the contents of your bodily waste. How uncomfortable it must be. Who really wants to know?

The medical staff standing above, giving medicines through the IVs that are in your arm; Propofol, that's a relaxation medication, oh, what about some Morphine that treats your pain and respiratory distress. Are you still with me? You can hear them talking over you, but you can't speak. You can blink, but unable to give directions. I'm sure you would want your input about what care you want to be stopped or continued. Again, you can't. Your family is standing at the bedside crying, deciding whether to make a decision to let you live or die. How do you feel as you read this? I'm having anxiety because I felt this several times over as I graced the halls of many ICUs; I envisioned myself being in one of those beds. I thank GOD this has never happened. The doctors are telling your family that you won't be the same Sam or Sarah they had known before you got sick. You won't be able to enjoy fried chicken, let alone eat a steak dinner. You have lost the ability to swallow food. Come closer, look at my eyes, what do you see? Am I not still here? Am I not a part of the conversation? Whose decision is it to say I will not recover? How are you feeling? What do you feel? I feel that if and when this ever happens to me, I want the best care, but most of all, my advanced directives will be written, and my family will only have to follow. Do you have yours done?

Goodbye Daddy... has been contemplated over a period until a recent tragedy struck in my life, as I began losing more of those I love and respect. I can hear their voices resonating in a whisper in my ears, "Beverly write your book!" Tell your stories; tell the people what your eyes have seen. Tell what day-to-day life is like working as a Social Worker; doing hospice, palliative care, home health, community advocate work, mediation and being a single parent. Tell those who will listen about the inevitable, the mental struggles of helping people. Share the drama the families have, along with the good and the bad, even though people may look at you strangely or may say, "Wow, your eyes have seen a lot." "People won't know what you've seen or done until you tell their stories and speak for them. You know of their life encounters, heartbreaks, heartaches, etc. What your eyes have seen and mind has experienced, will fail you one day; before they do, tell someone how this profession has impacted your life. Tell them how doing this work makes you wonder why GOD has chosen you to do what you do; interacting with families, seeing all this depressing stuff, because sometimes it is. As much as what you will say might hurt some, it's the truth. While telling their stories, tell yours." Open your heart; this is what Ms. Jo Lena, my publisher, has pressed and pushed. Tell the people how your eyes are your assets as they too tell the story behind your sadness, rejection, insecurities and shortcomings. Speak like no tomorrow about what you have seen.

I've encountered so many challenges with who I am internally, and prejudicially, because my skin tone is dark. Yes, I have several letters behind my name. That doesn't define me as a person, but it plays a major role in getting the ideal job I want and in garnering respect with other professionals, especially when holding crucial conversations. It's never easy, however. The shade of my skin is irrelevant, period. The question should be, *Are you equipped for the job?*

I've also seen and witnessed the heartache of families struggle with trying to decide what to do for their loved ones. As a medical social worker with 16 years of direct experience and 20 years of working in the community, I applied myself and graduated from St. Louis University with a Master's in Social Work, University of Missouri-St. Louis with a Master's Graduate Certificate in Non-Profit Management in Leadership along with a Bachelor's from Fontbonne University with a double minor in psychology and sociology. Let me give highest regards to where this education started, in 1989 at Forest Park Community College. I graduated in 1992 with an Associate Degree in Applied Science in Human Service and a Certificate in Gerontology. I don't know about you, I've earned my way. I'm coming before my readers to tell these stories and experiences speaking on behalf of the patients which will remain nameless to protect what will be said. Each of these stories are true accounts. I've gotten permission to tell the stories, but I'm electing not to say their names.

I have my own shortcomings as a social worker; by the time this book is published I pray that the licensure I'm seeking, that I've failed several times over, will have come to pass with an LMSW behind my name. I strive to work hard to show myself approved; the only one that approves all is GOD.

Goodbye Daddy addresses trust issues which I've encountered while working with families. While many caregivers are loving, sacrificing servants, many have been blamed for their wrong doings, like mismanagement of funds. Unfortunately, some keep their loved ones alive to collect a monthly check and keep them vented, but dead, to take care of financial business, selfishly. I have seen families dictate from the phone exhorting their power, only hurting their loved one who remains unresponsive and lifeless. Being a caregiver is an honor and should be treated as such. The life of a loved one is priceless. That's what believe and live by, doing this type of work.

"How much do you really value your loved one?" Is the question I ask my families and friends who are experiencing life-altering decisions. I also tell them, "No one is allowed to die because the process of leaving this earth is compromised too often with greed, negotiation and selfish gain. It shouldn't be that way." I hope my words encourage people to make responsible choices, without overstepping my bounds.

End Of Life Wishes Are Important

Have you considered what you want to happen to your material possessions and who you trust to manage them and your health in the event you cannot? Please consider what is important to you and share your wishes sooner rather than later.

"Let me go," are my wishes if I can't be Beverly. I'm that woman who wants to be remembered for the spirit of independence, love, compassion and heart. As I tell you their stories, I'm also telling my family mine. My mother, Lottie, my daughter, Desiray, my brothers, Chris and James and my niece Charlene, please don't compromise my life if I have an incurable disease and no further treatment is warranted or will help me sustain life.

Hospice is an excellent option when available. I love hospice and I support it fully as I understand the benefits it provides. Use it. If my care gets to be too much, put me in a nursing home, but one of those "five-stars" where they really look out for people. Make sure I'm bathed daily with my teeth brushed and put my smell good on me. Make sure I have that eye candy to keep my spirits alive. ⊠

Shackled Til Death..

— ❁ —

"He was days from dying, of no physical threat, as he lay on a ventilator, shackled by the ankles to his hospital bed."

Seven years of crying out, "I'm hurting, I'm hurting. I'm bleeding, I'm bleeding, please help me," all the while being ignored and going untreated is what lead Phillip to my floor in the hospital, following surgery for colon cancer.

As his mother, Ms. P, told me the events which led to Phillip's last stop, I could imagine the words, the sentiments and the feelings within him, all pent up, needing to be expressed:

"Momma, I'm sorry. Momma, please forgive me. I know I disappointed you and my kids. I hurt you all too much. I lived by these streets; I will die by these streets. I did what I had to do... But Momma, they don't care about me. They wouldn't listen to me. They own me, Momma. This is it. I love you, Momma. It's

good to be close to you again. I hope you can feel what I'm saying to you, Momma. Thank you for praying for me Momma."

His fellow inmates had to carry him when he could no longer walk up or down the prison steps to see the infirmary doctor. For seven years he'd been telling the prison guards that he's been bleeding from his penis and rectum. In each bowel movement Phillip had, he was bleeding out. Yet, nothing was done. What do you do when you are the property of the Federal Correctional System? "They don't care," are the words uttered from the mouth of his mother. All that matters is to "control the animal," which Phillip had been depicted to be. He didn't ask for this illness, nor did he have control over it. Rightfully so, his mother was angry as she expressed, "They could have treated him, isn't that what you and I, the taxpayers are paying for while these men and women are incarnated?"

I did my best to reassure her that we cared and we would do what we could to help her son, now. She replied, "His care *here* has been phenomenal," looking over her glasses beyond the long locs draping each side of her head. Watching her consumed with sadness, looking at a son she didn't recognize, I ached too. Tubes were everywhere, including a breathing tube and several lines of medication going into his body intravenously.

Seeing her son in this state turned her world upside down. I felt more like the warden's assistant than the social worker because I had to check in daily concerning all movements with their prisoner. *Yes sir, yes ma'am, he slept through the night, and his urine output was blah, blah, blah... Wait a minute! I don't work for you!* I immediately put a halt to that behavior and informed them that my nurse would give reports as things got complicated-medically. With his current state, things were deteriorating quickly and he was the priority, not the reports.

Ms. P explained:

"He sold drugs; he was in those streets being the man he was. His mentality was, 'Man who don't work, don't eat.' Slightly twisting the intent of the words of our parents and ancestors who stood firm on those principles. Well, Phillip did what he felt he had to do to feed his family. He sold that poison to his sisters and brothers who lived that lifestyle of getting high... In the end, he gained what by selling drugs? Doing what he needed to do landed him in prison, serving time, more than once. After all, who was going to hire a two-time convicted felon? The system isn't set up for those once convicted to obtain gainful employment. Once released, labeled a felon, on your record."

As she spoke, I was reminded of my cousin who was caught up in a revolving door of street life, jail and prison until his crimes got so severe that he is now serving two consecutive life sentences for violent crimes I dare not name. Even if he got out, who would hire him as a felon? They won't even consider him. His application would be considered a "File 13," trash. Where is their "clean-reform" opportunity act? Non-existent. Perhaps that's why Phillip was in those streets hustling? Selling drugs, and whatever else to make money to feed his family? Between all that selling, he managed to have four babies produced from two or three relationships until he got caught. What a shame, four more kids without a father, with the system taking care of them.

Social Working Through The Federal System

Our lives were now intertwined. I felt as though I was working for my cousin, on his behalf, as I saw the results of Philip's life, or the last of it, in my hands. It was a lot of work, complicated by the red tape of bureaucracy and the realities of criminalization in our society. Doing right by people who have made wrong choices is not easy, but it's what we must do.

I worked as the warden, the mediator, the voice, all the while being a support to Ms. P as she would soon lose her son, as his life expectancy was very short because of his complex medical problems. Phillip had metastatic liver and lung disease, he was on life support for acute respiratory failure and had a bullet in his stomach which had never been removed. When I read his kidney report, all kinds of stuff went through my head; this man was walking around with a bullet in his abdomen; *Who lives like this and survives? Was he that dude who didn't care? Was he that cocky or just that stubborn, continuing to be the drug dealer who got shot and survived? Why didn't he stop when he was given a chance at living?* I wasn't judging. My upbringing was around guys in the game selling drugs, carrying guns and by all means, making dirty money to come up to get what they wanted for cars, jewelry or simply feeding their families. Some guys/gals were smart enough to get in the game, make that money and get out. But most people know the game - if a person gets shot and lives, it's a sign to get out. We assumed God was saying something; game over, the next time you won't be as lucky. Looking at Phillip, I just wondered how it could happen. *How could a man be so young and so ill?* In prison, he began listening to his body, but because of the choices he made, he couldn't get the care he needed.

Ms. P shared that Phillip was very well-liked by the guys who were on lockdown with him. They became good friends and homeboys - they took care of each other. After all, everyone was spending years behind bars for their wrong doings. Their mindset was, "Might as well make good of what we have." She was grateful for them because they helped him once he was so frail. He would call home several times a week and then several times a day; his cellmate would call for him when he was too weak to do it himself. He told his mother that he was sick and the "people" didn't pay him any mind. Nurse after nurse, he told he was bleeding. Nurse after nurse, he told of the pain which had become so unbearable. Nurse after nurse, he was ignored and disregarded.

Phillip was slowly dying and didn't even know it. It wasn't until several calls from his mom to the correctional facility that his health concerns were taken seriously. One particular nurse saw him and knew he was sick and not faking his symptoms. She assessed him and knew he needed care beyond being in the infirmary. It was then Phillip was transferred to a local hospital in St. Louis. As is the protocol for Federal prisoners, he was shackled all the way there though he was in a semi-conscious state. When I saw him shackled to the bed, with two guards standing over him at all times, I thought of the movie, *Roots*.

Being Phillip's Social Worker

1) **Day One:** Phillip, 37-year-old, single, African-American, male with four children. Problem: We need a decision maker, other than the infirmary nurse for this patient, who is on mechanical life support. I made countless calls to get approval for patient's mother to be the decision maker while her son was in the hospital. Permission granted. Mother was called and a meeting was scheduled with her to discuss patient's status. Mother gave me full permission to do what was favorable for her son. Asked for shackles to be removed. Denied.

2) **Day Two:** Mother wants approval for patient's siblings and children to see their father. I made several calls and restrictions were set. Permission granted for children and sister to visit. Awaiting approval for patient's brother. Petitioned prison captain to get shackles removed so adequate care with dignity can be had. Message was left for this request.

3) **Day Three:** Sitting with patient's mother, as she shares her son's story, through voice trembles and hidden tears. The children were approved to come along with their mothers. The brother's request is still on hold. Shackle removal request denied again.

4) **Day Four:** Things are looking grim. We are scheduling to remove patient from the ventilator. I asked again for the removal of the shackles considering the medical state of the patient. He's dying, he's not a threat to get up and run. Request was denied a third time. One of the doctors spoke directly to the prison captain, after I did, requesting shackle removal. Tears filled the doctor's eyes as he was denied. Annie's Hope, the organization which focuses on supporting children whose family members are passing/have passed, was called for support. They came out to do palm prints of patient for his children as a memory of their dad. All children arrived and spent time with their dad. The waiting room was filled with family, most of whom were not on the approved list. Things started to get chaotic. Security was called to get order. Patient still shackled.

5) **Day Five:** Breathing tube was removed. Patient held his own for breathing but never awakened. I asked who will take the body once patient expires. Federal Correctional Facility provided me with details. They will take on the expense and remove the patient's remains. If patient's family wants a funeral, the family will incur the cost. His mother had to sign off on his body and that would be her last time physically touching her son. As the social worker, I called the funeral home to see if they would perform

a funeral once the body was released, they said yes. We discussed the cost and I shared that with the mother, who raised the additional amount necessary to have a service because she did not want her last memory of her son to be the one in that bed. Shackles remain.

6) **Day Six:** Patient was moved to a comfort suite in the hospital where his family could visit and spend his last hours and days. Support was provided. I spent time with the family and specifically with the patient's mother including hugs and conversation, as the grieving process had begun. At this point, she knew she was losing her son. Shackles and guards remain.

7) **Day Seven:** 6/11/16 at 6:32 am patient expired and transitioned this life. At the time of his death, my nurse requested, "Please can you take the shackles off, he's dead, he won't be going anywhere."

This journey was one of the most difficult in my career. Providing patient care while dealing with the devastating effects of long-term incarceration and family dynamics was heartbreaking. Thinking of Ms. P losing her son and her grandchildren now being fatherless is beyond sad.

*Dying shackled? I still think of **Roots**, and present day generational challenges, with limited options for freedom based on choices. The shackles remain.*

Flesh And Spirit

— ❧ —

"Morphine, when administered properly, acts as a pain medication and also calms breathing when a patient is in respiratory distress."

Dispelling myths is one of the biggest opportunities I have when dealing with families and their loved ones at the end of life. It's difficult to put the loved one's needs before the family's desires and wishes, especially when the time is short. People often resist certain treatments or options because of what they have heard. Other times, they make faith-based statements which tend to serve them versus being objective about the care and concern of their loved one. Or they have misinterpreted what they think are signs of faith because of limited perspective, fear of loss or they believe in a miracle which in many cases, is unrealistic by the time the loved one has reached the palliative or hospice care stage.

Denying pain medication, especially at the end of life is one of the cruelest things a person can do to a loved one yet, it happens too often when family members are "waiting on a miracle" from God to give them direction. This happened rather recently with a patient, Mr. Parker. To put it in context, have you ever heard the story about the flood? A flood happened and people went on their roof to "wait on God." A boat and a helicopter came to pick them up and they refused, saying God was going to rescue them, never attributing the boat and helicopter as being sent by God. Eventually, they died and when they got to heaven, God told them he had tried to rescue them, but their tunnel vision wouldn't allow them to make choices which would have resulted in being rescued in life, rather than in heaven. It's a sad, yet ironic story. And it's so similar to what I encountered with Mr. Parker's daughters, both pastors, who were charged with making decisions for their beloved father.

"Our faith is strong." "We know God's got this." "Our father is a man of faith who has equipped our family to believe and trust God for everything." Those are the words I constantly hear with boldness, trickle out the mouths of people of faith. I dare not dispute the power of God; I have experienced Him in my personal life, and I have seen His work through and with many families and friends. He's real. And, believing in God should not mean denying the obvious. *How long does one have to suffer before you are willing to let go and have a sense of peace about it? What will it take for the natural eye to see that the inevitable is near while allowing dignity with comfort to occur for the person who is dying?* God is real… what I'm saying is, why not allow the flesh and spirit to interact on mutual ground for decision making?

Yolanda and Gracie are two God-fearing pastors who preach, live and breathe by the spirit that dwells within; in this case, it is "GOD." It's no secret; they reverence God to the fullest believing that God will answer them, with the ability to discern their father's thoughts while listening to the aggressive medical staff who see struggle and pain. Rumbles of, "We're going to honor his wishes, when he no longer recognizes us or can speak, that's when we will shift gears and give him a medical remedy for comfort." The problem? Their father was in an extreme amount of pain and discomfort. Instead of allowing him medication, especially after chest surgery, they were "waiting for a sign" to say it was okay to give him morphine.

Mr. Parker was diagnosed with an aggressive form of lung cancer along with other medical problems which have debilitated him to being bedbound. He is a man of few words, because, in his current state, it exhausts him to talk. Prior to entering this final life's journey, he was active, very involved with the church, married for 50+ years to his high school sweetheart, and he was loving on his four children and a host of family and friends. In this particular case, Mr. Parker allowed his daughter, his favorite as I was told, to be his voice. I had my reservations about this and wondered why his wife wasn't making these decisions. Mrs. Parker, a retired nurse herself, was filtered information by Yolanda and Gracie during their visits. It was quite strange. Once the information was provided, they made a collective decision to either pursue treatment or not.

Mr. Parker was so challenged that he could barely breathe on his own. It was explained that the procedure needed was risky, a chest tube, to pull some of the fluid from his lungs. He made it through the surgery and then he was to wear a Bi-PAP mask to blow the forced air through his lungs. A Bi-PAP is a non-invasive mechanical pressure support ventilation which gives positive airway pressure. Rather than having a tube down your throat to breathe for you, you have a mask on your face blowing constant air to help you breathe. Many patients complain that it is annoying. Mr. Parker feels the same way and no longer wants the Bi-PAP to help him breathe.

Though the daughters wanted him to keep wearing it, they begrudgingly honored his wish and we removed the mask. Immediately, as expected, his breathing became challenged. The staff pleaded with them to be given permission to administer a small dose of morphine through the IV to lessen his symptoms of air hunger. "Did you know that morphine, can relax him, so he's not struggling for air?" is what I said. "Oh, but he can't have it…" is what the daughter said. She explained, "The family wants him conscious and aware. They say that morphine will speed his death up and make him more sleepy." *Who is they, I wonder?* We explain that without the morphine, he's going to die quicker, within an hour or so, because of his symptoms and the disease process. They refused the morphine saying, "Our father dictated through spirit that he doesn't want the morphine." I can't say what's true for them, but I can speak to the myth.

This myth of morphine has plagued the African-American community for years on end. I have found it to be a struggle at times explaining the positive effects of morphine in that it aids in the pain management of symptoms while assisting with the struggle of experiencing air hunger.

I know it's difficult to let go, especially when you are raised as a God-fearing person and what you want may not align with the actual medical condition of a loved one. However, recognizing that non-emotional, objective decisions need to be made during highly emotional times, especially when a loved one is suffering is crucial and necessary. Accepting God's will may look and seem different than "saving" a loved one in the final hour.

Speaking from my own heart and experience, we never want to let them go, however, trusting that if they are going, knowing it is bigger than us, can help with the grieving process.

The Incomplete Stroke

— ✿ —

"Strokes tend to take away important parts and pieces..."

She is a mother and a published fiction writer who expresses herself without any mental or physical limitations; until it happened...

"Where's my voice? I can't move my legs... my arms? Oh Lord, I'm paralyzed. My work is incomplete. My thoughts, my book, my living... Not now! This can't be happening. My dear and faithful son, who will see after you? Lord, I know you have the answers to this tragedy but who will explain this journey for me? Son, if you trust and believe in our GOD, this is your test, people will watch and see if you will honor me as the scripture says. Are you equipped son to endure this walk? Hello, I'm in here; talk to me son. Son? Son! Oh no, he can't hear me. I can't hear me. I have no voice..."

I was on the phone, talking with my sister when my speech started to slur. I remember her asking if I was okay. I couldn't fully comprehend what she was saying, but I knew something was wrong, I felt it; this intense traveling pain going up my arm, and along came the numbness of my face, arm and leg; the phone dropped first. I attempted to stay up, but my balance was off; down to the floor I went. I lay helplessly on the kitchen floor. I could see the phone. It was out of reach. My son was at work. I tried yelling. Something was wrong. My voice was not working. Fortunately, my sister's call had not disconnected when the phone fell from my hands. She heard me go down and called 911.

"Hello, I'm in here, talk to me, tell me what's happening. I see my son crying; no words uttered just cries of hurt and pain. Lying helplessly on my back, I see that bright light. Ouch! No... do not stick me! That hurts. Oooh, please stop. What's wrong with you? I told you I'm in here, I just can't answer. It's dark, the light is fading, I can't breathe..."

"My life is not done. I am not finished. Look into my eyes, can you read them? Son, do you hear me?"

Everything is incomplete. Breathing tubes, IVs, medications being pushed into her veins, machines singing in harmony. Is this new life for her? The incomplete stroke has left her debilitated and having to be cared for 24 hours a day, seven days a week.

"What kind of suffering is this? I would rather you let me go than look down upon me daily, being a burden. Where is the exit sign?..."

"Honor your father and your mother, as
the LORD your God has commanded you, so that
you may live long and that it may go well with
you in the land the LORD your God is giving you.
Deuteronomy 5:16 (NIV)

Lost Treasures

—— ❀ ——

"I changed your diapers and put you through school, and you throw me into a nursing home because you can't stand the smell of me?"

"What's that smell?!? Is that feces on my white diamond Berber carpet? Who's cleaning that up?

My walls are supposed to be white! Why are they stained with fingerprints? What the hell is going on, can't you see?

I'm tired of washing clothes multiple times a week that reek of urine! OMG, I have to throw up.

Look at these scratches and scrapes along the walls and door entrances from that walker! Woman, get somewhere and sit down!

I'm hoarse because you can't hear me! You need to wear those hearing aids! Oh, yes, I didn't get you any..."

Plagued with voices which speak inside her head, she refuses to take her medications or eat; and falsely accuses people of spitting in her food. Ms. Claire just needs some TLC and a couple of clothing protectors. An adult diaper to catch the urine, and an adult bib or even big towel will do just nicely.

"I'm around all these strangers and it stinks in here! I was born and raised in the south with no formal education, became a widow after my last child was born when a drunk driver hit my husband, who died on impact.

Where is my family? I've worked my ass off to make sure my kids were cared for and had the best of everything. Yes, four children were raised to success by the blood and sweat I endured; where are those grown children now? Where's Mary Beth, Nurse Practitioner? Where's Logan, Defense Attorney? Where's Abigail, Geriatrician? Where's Scott, Renowned Motivational Speaker?"

They all drove cars whose names she couldn't pronounce, with homes that you would only see in a magazine, but she's tossed away in a nursing home. What did she do to deserve such injustice? She may forget things; pee on herself a time or two, and even make a mess trying to feed herself, but she has all her faculties. Who lives to be 90, with everything working the way it used to, nobody!?!

"Why was I put in a nursing home? Why can't I be with my family?"

Those are the words I've heard from Ms. Claire and others time and time again. Repeatedly successful children are not compassionate enough to take care of the hand that fed them, but instead, throw them away in a room shared by a total stranger.

Six Considerations Prior To Nursing Home Placement

There comes a time when caring for a loved one is too difficult. Instead of just "throwing them away" without explanation, sharing what's happening, why it's happening, and being part of their lives, regardless of where they live is crucial to health and well-being.

1. Accept that you can't take care of your loved one.
2. Sit down and talk to them about what's going on and why.
3. Explore options for nursing home placement. Perhaps let them walk around with you, taking a tour and seeing how they may adjust.
4. Once placement happens, make sure it's as homelike as possible. Small things like including favorite pillows, decorations or treasured items such as photos help.

5. Visit regularly and always tell them you love them at the end of each visit.
6. Don't feel guilty about making the placement especially if it is in the best medical interest of your loved one.

Too many times I've seen greed and selfishness outweigh elderly care decisions. Be good to your relatives and be willing to treat them at least as good as you treat yourself.

Goodbye Daddy

Dual Roles

— ❀ —

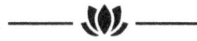

"Being the social worker and the niece was heart-wrenching."

As a hospice social worker, I deal with families every day, as they are dealing with critical illnesses and anticipated loss. When my aunt was placed on hospice, it was difficult for me because I wasn't really prepared to need the love and assurances I often give others, during those delicate moments close to her passing.

My family requested me to be the social worker in my aunt's case. Due to the circumstances, my employer allowed it. In one sense, I was happy to serve in that role, because I wanted to make sure her needs and concerns were addressed. On the other hand, I wondered how performing dual roles would affect me, and how I would navigate through the process. She was my favorite aunt, after all.

It was tough. I've often said that the Lord won't put more on me than I can bear. That's a true statement, yet when I carry the burdens of others, it is easier to do. The families find comfort because I have my relationship with God. The only way I can truly be of service to them is because of Him. I give Him their burdens once they've been passed to me. They don't know, in those moments, comfort, resources and relief are what matters. When it was time to carry my burdens, with the pain of seeing my aunt transition before my eyes, I had to give Him the weight because He was the one who kept me upright, as I had many moments I was ready to fall.

Day one was a struggle; navigating the unimaginable anticipated grief. In my 20 plus years of healthcare and 12 years as a hospice social worker, this was the closest case to my heart and home.

As the days passed, sitting for hours on end at the door, waiting to "go home" is all she spoke about. Her mind wasn't healthy anymore as the voices talked to her. My Auntie was so beautiful, with flawless skin, pearly white straight teeth, and long grayish/blue tinted hair. My cousin who is a beautician kept her hair fixed.

Auntie was a caring, giving, faithful servant in the church and matriarch of her family. I saw the slow decline right before my eyes, but I was in denial; I knew what the end results would be; I'd seen this too many times with other patients. She was very sick with heart and kidney issues. Auntie had lots of swelling in her hands and ankles which looked like little puff balls.

No pain, but much tightness is what she would say when asked, "How do your hands feel?" She never complained, but I still hear the words resonating in my mind; "When am I going home?" I knew this meant one of two things; transitioning or wanting to go to a place where she once lived. In this case, at that moment, it was going back to a familiar place, and it was her home with her son. My dearest aunt stayed coherent until her last few days of life.

Before I tell you about her last moments, I want you to know that she was loved dearly by me. She was at my wedding, dressed to impress; and gave me her blessings even though my marriage only lasted three years, she knew I loved him since I said I do... Anyway, I've moved on to happier living... I saw my aunt as a woman of status, poise and grace. She always gave me words of wisdom and spoke of the Lord and His goodness which is upon my life. She would give me words of encouragement when she felt my spirit was empty. Don't mistake her, Auntie held her own very well and would check you with words and looks telling you it was time to get your stuff together. I was often checked when I saw her.

Auntie was a classy, hat wearing, sophisticated, woman who was extremely well-dressed. Little did Auntie know she gave me what most young women seek from their mothers, validation. Validation that whatever I desired, God loved me enough to listen; she reminded me to pray and ask God and she assured me He would answer. And by example she showed me most of all, to "be a woman and carry yourself as such." She validated me as being a beautiful, smart woman who could conquer anything once God is acknowledged in it.

I loved when I was a little girl seeing her at church with the finest white dress suits and matching hats; she was the sharpest dressed mother in the church. No other mother could touch her style. I believe this is where I get my love of wearing hats, as my mother doesn't wear them.

Auntie had a good life; she was married to my uncle who I felt was the "best man" any woman would love to have. See, I recognized what love was at a young age, watching them. Uncle was a good father, provider and man of God who walked upright; faultless in my eyesight and many others. I can't say that about most men I've encountered, there's fault amongst us, but again, I say what I perceived to be love, honesty and the care that a woman is destined to have from her man; they don't make them like that anymore. When Uncle got sick, Auntie took good care of him. He professed his love until he took his last breath. Unfortunately, Uncle transitioned life years before Auntie took ill. As she lived her life without Uncle, her supporting family was there. She has two beautiful daughters and two sons, one of which preceded her in death. The family was so supportive, you would have thought that there wasn't a loss. The family kept Uncle's legacy of love alive as if he never left.

Years later, Auntie needed to downsize from that huge home in which she was living. Her daughters and son assisted in preparing her for the move. During this time, Auntie started showing signs that something was wrong; frequent hospitalization with blood pressure issues, unexplained swelling in both her legs along pronounced hand/arm swelling and memory problems. Thank God her children and grandchildren were attentive enough to know that something wasn't right. Each time Auntie would go to the doctor, family and church members always showed up and out in attendance. They truly loved my aunt.

"When am I going home?"

"Could you call and find out when I'm leaving this place? Did they leave me here to die?" Is all she talked about during each one of our encounters. Each visit I would call my mother to let her know I

was with her sister. Even though it hurt my mother to her soul that her sister was in a nursing home, I had to explain to her, the reason why, as she like neighbors, church members and others objected to the choice.

Unfortunately, people don't understand that when a person's care gets beyond what they can handle in the home, they have to rely on more experienced folks with 24-hour care in place. Auntie needed nursing home placement. I won't dwell on the mad folks who felt my cousin could have taken my aunt home with her; my cousin suffers from crippling rheumatoid arthritis and she needed assistance. With her mother's level of care, this would have been a failure all the way around if she was to take my aunt home with her. There was another daughter, but she lived out-of-town. She frequently visited Auntie; every opportunity she had. Every opportunity they took Auntie home for the weekend, but it was difficult when she returned; she wouldn't get out of the car making it almost impossible even to consider taking her out again. What a chore and what heartache it was to see this.

One particular day Auntie wasn't right; she was having a conversation with "the voices." Once inside her room to visit, she wouldn't let me leave. She used her body to barricade the door. When I tried to leave, she would tell me, "No!" "No, you're not going anywhere!" I was frightened because I recognized this was not my aunt. When I would try to move her, she let me know not to put my hands on her. She also spoke of my brother being outside the room trying to harm her. At that moment I knew my aunt was experiencing some form of delusions. This captivity took about 45 minutes of asking and pleading to let me out the room. It wasn't until I switched roles from the niece to the social worker, and I spoke in a firm, but aggressive tone that she "came back."

Using the professional tone hurt me to speak to my aunt this way, but the "sweet pleading niece" had been totally disregarded for nearly an hour. When I spoke as the social worker, she listened. I told her in a firm voice, "You will move from this door and you will not harm me." Auntie looked at me and said, "You ain't leaving either." It wasn't until I spoke again in a calm, aggressive tone that she moved from the door and sat down on the bed.

That day changed my life. I asked God, "How can a God-fearing woman who served Him faithfully hear voices?" I was overcome with a profound sense of sadness. I had to walk out of the nursing home to get myself together. I exited the facility and found myself in my car crying as if someone took the life out of me; in this case, I saw the "beginning of the end" with my aunt. At that moment, I asked God to help me because I knew one of these roles would suffer.

I visited my aunt every week until I couldn't separate the roles. I would go in as a social worker weekly; if I didn't do anything else, I would read the Bible, polish her nails or comb her hair. I was at her bedside; I was there listening to her talk to someone, only visible in her mind. She would even say to me, "I'm not crazy," accepting that the voices were speaking to her in her head.

As time passed, Auntie would just nod at the voices; she was feeling some way since I knew they were there. She would stay in bed at the request of the voices telling her to stay put. When I say I was through in the natural as being a niece, my feelings couldn't bear it any longer. Although I had to be the social worker to deal with this situation, the niece was still there in the background suffering.

I supported the family as decisions were made regarding putting Auntie on dialysis. They had hope that doing so would extend her life. Based on her symptoms, I knew the journey would end quickly. However, my cousins did not ask my opinion about the dialysis, the dementia and heart failure. It's a lethal combination, as dialysis weakens the heart and dementia prevents patients from making sound judgment. Yet, I had no authority/opinion technically in Auntie's care. If this was a normal case, with people who were not my relatives I'm sure they would have been more open to my expertise and knowledge, asking for my professional opinions and options for care.

June 23, 2016, was the last time I interacted with my aunt. I was able to spend time with her; just me and her. She allowed me to do her fingernails after eating a few chips to her delight. I put a beautiful coat of burgundy polish on them; she thought she was at the nail salon; that's how nice I did them. Who knew that would have been my last day interacting with my aunt? What I did know was, I had a hurting sensation in my heart that I couldn't explain. I saw that she was leaving me but I was blinded in this dual role; the niece did not want to see her go.

When we lost Auntie, my cousin and her husband said, "Beverly, I know she was your favorite aunt. It's okay to cry," the tears flooded down my cheeks as I released the pain of loss, grateful to grieve freely as the niece.

Auntie, you are missed.

Your smile was my motivation to keep waiting on God for all my everlasting needs. Thank you for loving me and giving me the word of GOD to keep reaching for unlimited adventures. I thank my family for allowing me to tell this story. I thank Pastor Tate at Olivette Missionary Baptist Church for that powerful eulogy: The Irreversible Commodity.

Auntie will never be duplicated and neither will we ever have a do over.

A Dedicated Veteran

— ❧ —

"Thanks for your service."

Diagnosed in 2013, Mr. Peterson had a radical cystectomy with ileostomy (that's the removal of the entire bladder, nearby lymph nodes, part of the urethra with a stoma, where the urine will go into a special bag called a urostomy pouch). He had multiple rounds of chemotherapy treatments to combat this disease. However, it returned with a vengeance, and more aggressively in December 2015.

By August 2016, when he became my patient, he had a severe case of thrush, a non-contagious infection which accumulates in the mouth. His tongue and cheeks were completely white coated; how painful, I thought.

I witnessed Mrs. Peterson as she touched her husband only slightly, because of his frailty, afraid of the anticipated pain she may cause. The look of anguish in her eyes spoke volumes - I felt her pain of hurt with disappointment. Looking down at her husband as he lay helplessly in the hospital bed, dependent on people for his every need; bathing, medication, turning, feeding, how dehumanizing. Mr. Peterson served this country, and all Mrs. Peterson wanted was the preservation of the good times, joy and affection they shared.

This former soldier was suffering greatly. Mr. Peterson had hypertension, stage 4 urothelial cell carcinoma, (bladder cancer) and he was stricken with type 2 diabetes, along with kidney failure and extensive liver lesions. At times he was able to answer simple questions with a yes or no. However, he also had dementia, which clouded his clarity and ability to reason. He was able to converse, but only at a whisper accompanied by a simple nod of yes or no. Plagued with so much, it was difficult to see him living his final days, suffering in pain. I needed to know his last wishes, if at all possible.

Day 4

(Phone ringing)
Hello. Mrs. Peterson, this is Beverly, the social worker from the hospital, is this a good time to talk?

(Agitated)
"I'm at work, what is it you want?' I have to get back
to what I'm doing, and I have to stay focused, and
why are you calling me? Is everything alright with
my husband?

(Calmly)
Ma'am, if I may, I need a minute of your time to
schedule a family meeting to discuss goals of care
and treatment options for Mr. Peterson.

(Sighing with annoyance)
What are you saying? He's doing well, isn't he? Tell
me he's okay! I just left him…

(Calmly)
Ma'am, please calm down… if you can just take a
moment, I'm really sorry to upset you; that's not
why I called.

(Voice becomes weak, still annoyed)
What is it?!?…

(Calmly)
Mrs. Peterson, I would prefer not to tell you this
over the phone, and would rather sit down with
you, along with our team and provide options.

(Angry and scared)
Just tell me... tell me! What do you want? I can't take any more of the late night calls about him not being able to breathe! So. What. Do. You. WANT? What Ms. Beverly do you want?

(Calmly)
Your husband has a limited life expectancy, and I want to know how he would want it to transpire?

(Short sigh)
I'm sorry. You don't deserve this. I love him. I want him to live. I know he doesn't have much time, but I need more time with him.

(Calmly)
I endure this every day as a social worker. At first, people see me as the enemy, but I'm here to help. I'm so sorry that any of my families have to go through this. I know this is tough and I'm here to hold your hand. So it's okay. Let me help you, please...

(She interrupts)
I don't want my husband to return to this nursing home. He was here for three months. His health declined so rapidly. I'm overwhelmed being his wife and caretaker. I thought to bring him to where I work, would allow me to spend more time while keeping my eyes on him while I work. I thought I could trust my coworkers to do their jobs and take care of him. They didn't care at all.

(Calmly)

Yes, Mrs. Peterson, trying to be in dual roles is tough, I tried it, and it doesn't work. It's too easy to run yourself into the ground. That's why I'm calling, to offer my support. If you let me support you, perhaps we can get him much better care, together?

(More calmly)

Okay. A Veterans Home is where I would like him to go. He deserves dignity, and to be treated with respect and care. He is a Veteran after all. He dedicated his life serving our country. I think he would want that too.

(Calmly)

Thank you. I'll be glad to work on that. Just as I was assigned to your husband's case, I'm here for you, too.

(Mumbling weakly)

Why can't we preserve his life, just for a little while?

It was clear that she was conflicted. I could tell her initial annoyance was overshadowing her anxiety. Her husband was extremely sick, yet she wanted him to live. To be preserved, somehow. She was shifting from wanting "it" over to wanting him "here." She didn't want him to suffer. I could relate to what she was thinking and feeling. In those moments, there's no real time to process; you just have to make decisions.

(Sniffling)
Mrs. Peterson said, "This can't be happening; he served his country, and now he's dying. What happened to honoring our Veterans for life?"

I felt bad for her, knowing that he did serve. I respect our Veterans and know they deserve every measure of care and support. I couldn't do much for him, in his condition. For the previous three months, he was at that nursing home, being neglected. Sad, indeed. I could tell by looking at his body. If only we could do more, like she wanted, in the snap of a finger.

(With more confidence)
Please move him, she said.
I worked to get Jefferson Barracks to accept him, and they did, that day, which is very rare, as they are often full, with a waiting list.

Day 5

Unfortunately, Mr. Peterson passed, before being transported early this morning. I say that was God working in the midst because Jefferson Barracks was a 45-minute drive from where the family lived and a daily commute would have been even more overwhelming for Mrs. Peterson after having worked an eight-hour day.

After his transition, I looked at his body and saw that he was bruised from arm to arm, not from the fault of the medical team, but from the results of blood tests, IVs, and having thin skin from aging and all of his ailments.

At ease soldier, you are now dismissed from your duties.

A Partner's Love

—— ❦ ——

"Jay Jay's life was crumbling down, and the family wanted nothing to do with him."

"Yeah, I'm gay, so is your daddy. Get over it. I've begged you to be here because I want to respect your dad's wishes and I'm hoping we can work it out. I can see your face and tell you don't want to be here. But the deal is, with or without you, I'm going to do right by your daddy. You being the prodigal son, you failed him with your ruthlessness and drug-using lifestyle. You've only seen him four times in four years, and that's only when you wanted something or were begging to get bailed out of trouble. But you sit at this round glass table with mounds of used snot tissues crying, not able to speak up when the social worker addresses you. Why in the hell are you mad? Look here Sonny Boy, what you fail to realize is when your daddy needed you, you left town on one of your tirades, very accusatory, abusive, and disrespectful. He needs you now. What are you going to do?"

Boisterous Bryan, Jay Jay's partner of 15 years, was certainly a character. A narcissistic, 375 pound, 6'2" extremely feminine gay man who had his own health issues, but I wasn't there to judge. I appreciated him caring enough to get Jay Jay's son to the hospital, and the way he was speaking up when my own voice was not being heard.

Jay Jay is a left-legged, below the knee amputee, who often experienced phantom pain. Bryan provided the most tender and gentle touch to his partner during my visit. Bryan rubbed Jay's stump as he consoled him lovingly. Jay Jay, with his eyes closed, seemed to bask in the adoration and attention as his body and fears were soothed by the one person who hadn't turned his back on him.

Jay Jay was married at one time, they had a boy child, pretty much setting this kid up for failure with giving him a girl's name, London. Jay Jay got tired of this cramped closet living, so he sprouting through the cracks, to be the full-fledged, proud gay man he is. I'm quite sure some of y'all are out here living double lives so please don't act shocked by my candor. I'm not here to judge. Just be happy and live life, it's too short to be compromised by those who make different choices. Jay Jay just refused to hide it any longer. He got divorced, and he took his first real breath of living, freely. Bryan stepped into Jay's life at a very critical time when they were only friends.

On this day, Bryan called him his blonde/grey super soulful, hot and spicy, sexy boo-thing among other descriptive and humorous adjectives. They provided each other with love, warmth, guidance, affection and all the trimmings any relationship desires. Jay had a void, and Bryan filled it. Bryan needed Jay to be his muse and audience. He allowed him to be colorful, adventurous and free to love life. Jay Jay never really met a stranger.

Jay Jay suffered his first stroke, which left him in a debilitated state, at the age of 56 and had kidney failure, which led him to receive dialysis. A few months later doctors told him that he had advanced lung cancer with spinal and pelvic metastases. Imagine getting a quadruple report of this nature?

I can't imagine. Seeing his frowned up face told me he's in pain. Pain was written all over him, every single movement. I hurt for him; no one wants to be young and stricken with such debilitating diseases, especially at a time where you're supposed to be enjoying life and having fun.

Jay Jay needed someone to care for him. He and Bryan had discussed, in detail, his wishes and Bryan did what he could to get the family involved. Bryan may have been his partner but Jay's family: sister, brother, parents and a son had cut him off because of his lifestyle. No one was willing to step up. It seemed that they had their own internal issues, knowing that Jay was a gay man who came out of the closet. You know how people get with their judgmental chants, "God's gonna kill you dead having sex with a man." Let any man or woman step forward who is without fault.

"Speak up London! What do you have to say?"

Bryan waited and waited for the voice of validation from Jay's son to no avail. When London failed to advocate for his dad, Jay told Bryan to seek legal guardianship over him. One evening London agreed to meet Bryan at a bar where he consumed five drinks. During his intoxicated tirade, London voiced his hurt, hate and the betrayal he felt from his father, all directed at Bryan. He wasn't going to help him get guardianship nor was he going to stop him, as he ended by saying, "Thanks for taking care of my dad." The next day Jay made Bryan promise him that he would take care of him no matter what the ugly faces of the world would say as they were judged about their sexual orientation.

Lying in bed, this withdrawn, frail man, who was unable to do for himself, continued to be comforted by Bryan's touch. Jay's thin face was unshaven, yet his fingernails were manicured to perfection, with both wrists draped with pink and white crystal, handmade bracelets. With his eyes closed, he asked for Jay's hands to rub his missing leg; he gently rubbed at each request. The genuine love they shared reminded me of love I once knew.

I'm glad Bryan and London got together over drinks though nothing got resolved for his father. I listened as Bryan relayed what was really happening with Jay Jay's son, through tears and sorrow. Bryan revealed what London was going through; he had lost custody of his son just two days prior, and his mother was dying in another state with similar issues as his father. How tragic and overwhelming all of this must have been for him. Hence, the heavy drinking and continued drug abuse. Not judging, he was coping the way he learned.

Jay Jay was discharged from the hospital and passed about eight days later.

"Love is love, no matter what. Respect it."

Unpacking Your Case

——— ❦ ———

Wanda's mother, Cutie, was 95 years old. Before becoming ill, she was full of life until her mind started doing things beyond her control. At 4'9", 75 pounds, her momma started cussing Wanda out, accusing her of stealing her money, all the while uncontrollably walking around urinating and defecating on herself. Wanda thought, *What the hell is this?* But she didn't do anything about it. Wanda had no clue that her mom had Alzheimer's. She was in denial. She wouldn't get the help needed for her mom, and the help her mother needed for herself. She didn't take things seriously until Cutie walked down the street aimlessly, naked. Thank goodness someone saw this frail, elderly little lady and called 911 before it got any worse.

Wanda rushed from work to the hospital's ER. Once there, Dr. D did his assessment and knew within minutes Cutie had Alzheimer's, a form of dementia. Wanda sat in a stoic manner at the bedside like Dr. D was speaking in a foreign language she did not understand or comprehend. "Wanda, Wanda, are you ok? Can you hear me?" Dr. D inquired. After moments of silence, Wanda pushed for speech, burst into tears and unexpectedly began crying out, pouring her thoughts, emotions and heavy burdens into the room. Screaming, yet not necessarily speaking directly to Dr. D she said, "What am I going to do? I have so much going on! I've isolated my mom from family, who's going to *help me*? I've been battling depression behind the murder of my son. I've been angry with my so-called friends and family who are more like enemies since they abandoned me. I have no clue as to what to do!"

As if the trance had lifted, she looked in his eyes and said, "Dr. D what am I going to do? I can't, I just can't do this. Do I put her in a nursing home? Oh, I can't the guilt will eat me up…" Dr. D called for the social worker to help. While waiting for the social worker to show, Dr. D asked about Cutie's life before her illness, along with how long Wanda had been in denial… as she responded it was clear, her suitcase was packed to overflowing.

Every day, all day, situations like these are what I am faced with as a healthcare professional. Families have so much going on with their own issues until they get overwhelmed and unable to make conscious decisions. Wanda is depressed, overwhelmed,

Goodbye Daddy

frustrated and understandably hurt behind losing a child. As a result, she has become self-isolated and removed Cutie from family and friends along with not dealing with her mental health and emotional issues. She, like many others had tried to handle things herself instead of seeking assistance when things became noticeably difficult for her and her mother.

Unfortunately, Wanda's concerns are very similar to most adults as we age. If it's not our parents or grandparents, it may be us, who need special care. The suitcases, while they may conceal many things for a time, cannot hide or hold everything.

What's in your suitcase?

A pressed white shirt? Two pairs of slacks? A straw Fedora hat? Brown leather loafers? Six pairs of underwear? Perhaps two pairs of socks? Three pairs of tights? Those traditional black heels with the polka dot bows? What else are you carrying? What's in the pockets? Depression, guilt, low self-esteem, insecurities, hurt? Anger, humiliation, shame, abandonment, pride, regrets? Is it too much? Yes, it's too much. Will your shoulder straps break? Yes, they will. When is enough, enough for you? Will you require a life-threatening episode before you realize that something is wrong? What will it take for you to accept support, guidance and maybe even forgiveness? Is stubbornness in your case too? It starts and ends with you.

A Free Mind Allows For Focus

Unpacking all that stuff frees your mind. Too many people, including entire families, exist daily, overwhelmed. The guilt of what they did or didn't do. Shame for not speaking or stepping up. Hiding behind secrets. Anger spirals up and down, creating situations out of their control. The weight of the bag, filled with its contents creates untreated wounds which become infected and irreversible if not addressed. The eyes say it all. Puffy, encircled, bloodshot... Trembling hands. Tapping toes. Avoiding contact... the wounds take over. You do have authority. You do have control.

Aren't you tired of your shoulders hurting from the straps which are allowing you to carry such baggage? Are you tired of cradling that suitcase like a football ready to score a touchdown?

How will you unpack your case?

As a social worker, I've taught families to unpack their cases, one issue at a time. It's important to take the most pressing matters and start with them, one day at a time, minute by minute, second by second until release and relief occur. If your issues include any of those above, explore where they are coming from, acknowledge them, talk about them with those who can do something about them, and keep going.

One method I highly recommend is journaling. Express on paper what is happening and why you think it. Then go on to explore how you feel about it all. When you write things down, your thoughts, feelings, emotions and regrets, this begins a healing process because you are no longer holding these things inside. It can also assist in communicating with others, your needs.

You can't do it all by yourself. Seeking wise counsel and professional care is critically important and can support you through. Then, tackle the next issue. If you are struggling to unpack the problems, perhaps more help is required. That's when social workers like me can assist in exploring resources, giving referrals, or recommendations to families.

I implore you to start unpacking those cases.
Otherwise, your straps will succumb and break.

Making A Wish Foundation

— ❧ —

"When we take the time to find a need, we can at times, do something to fulfill it."

On an unusually warm day in January, I was assigned to a Queen. Queen comes with a unique story to tell, as she is a woman of favor and grace. "I've buried my parents, all my aunts and uncles and five of the seven children I gave birth to," she said. When I say a woman of status with dignity and gratitude, you can't help but love her.

Queen is a 102-year-old, African American woman who lives in her senior apartment. Her grandchildren, Darnell, Mickey, and Jackie, are her caregivers seven days a week, around the clock. Queen has profound hearing loss, which requires writing down words to converse with her. Her grandson, she understands as she reads his lips when she is not able to understand what is written.

Humbled by her presence, I am honored to be talking with this matriarch of seven generations. I was speechless, after introducing myself to this beautiful display of longevity before me. I can truly say God has kept Queen's mind and she understands what is being said without being confused. She is a woman of soft beauty and sheer elegance with flawless, glowing skin. She had a reputation of being extremely generous, serving many, and being very kind.

During my visit to her home, I noticed a portion of Queen's legacy, including a framed letter of Proclamation from the Mayor of St. Louis when she turned 100 years old. Next to the letter was a picture of her proudly receiving the proclamation, dressed in an all-white, beaded dress suit with a matching beaded white hat featuring a beautiful bow. When I asked about this picture, Queen's eyes lit up, and she began to cry. I allowed the pause and the tears to flow, then I asked her grandson, Darnell, "Did I say something wrong?" His response was, "She's happy. People near and far showed up. It was standing room only." I asked glancing at the photo once more, "What would make her smile like that again?" Darnell informed me that they would be honoring their grandmother for the last hoorah before exiting this life and they were seeking to purchase another dress suit and hat. She adores the colors blue and pink.

This woman had done so much for everyone else; I wanted to do something important for her. As the assigned social worker, I asked for a monetary wish to be granted to purchase a dress suit for Queen's. This ceremony for acknowledgment was to be held in March at her church, Greater Bethel Baptist Church.

I applied to the Hospice Foundation for a gift to obtain a beautiful suit for Queen's ceremony honoring her life. They granted the wish and donated $600.00! She got the prettiest white laced, Donna Vinci rhinestone with an elegant white pearl lace trimmed two-piece dress suit, accented with a Donna Vinci hat, derby style with white lace trimming, she was so sharp. Hmmm, reminds me of my beautiful, classy aunt who wore dresses of this caliber; truly women of class. On this particular day, speakers from as far as Washington, D.C. came and acknowledged her works in the community with families and countless friends whose lives she impacted. Speaker after speaker spoke about her unselfish love and dedication that she spread across the states. Mayors, congressmen and women from St. Louis and her hometown in Clarksdale, Mississippi paid their respects. Kind words of what this beautiful, God-fearing woman's life entailed were expressed through songs and praise dancing.

What an endearing way to honor a Queen. I pray when I reach a dear sweet, ripe age, I too am remembered with love of that magnitude.

Four weeks later, at her homegoing, she rested in that beautiful suit. As we honored her life we smiled, knowing her spirit was flowing.

"Being able to do something for a woman who spent her life doing for others was one of the highlights of my career."

Hidden Secrets

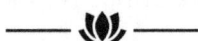

— ❀ —

"Secrets don't necessarily die at death."

He was a dirty old man. And he was her dirty old man. It didn't make it better, it was just true.

I noticed she wears her hair covering one eye. There's no sense of happiness inside of her. Our conversation started with the question, "How's your relationship? Have you always been connected or has there been a rift between you all? I'm asking because I see tears and I want to know what these tears mean." She was suicidal and said she had attempted to take her life three weeks ago. I immediately started praying with her out loud. I asked her why she was depressed, wanting to get to the root...

She told me that her grandmother sold her mother for sex. Then she said she forgives her father and mother. Then she shut down immediately. After a few moments, she shared with me that she was raped. She has an 8-year-old son who she treats like a baby. She protects him a lot. I said, "I know that's your baby…" and I shared how overprotective I was with my daughter, until one day she talked to me about it. The young lady listened to my story and then I added that she has to give him a bit of freedom saying, "Let him hang out with his friends and play. If you don't, it will harm him more so than help him."

He won't learn how to do certain things if she doesn't allow him to open up and have new experiences. She said she didn't want anything to happen to him like it happened to her. I told her I understood but that he had to be allowed to have friends and do things like sleep-overs. And even if she didn't trust other homes or parents, she could offer a safe-haven of her own for him and his friends, perhaps being able to support them, because she was opening her home to them.

Her darkness is full of thoughts of rape, how her mom was not the mother she thought she was, how she was taking care of her mother and father, and how inappropriate her father is, or at least was, before the stroke.

He would regularly show her photos on his phone of other women's body parts. He even went so far as to tell her 10-year-old daughter that he has a penile implant! When she said that, my eyes bucked. She said she was so serious. He was such an attention seeker that he would say just about anything to get attention from just about anyone. After she told me that, she began to tell me that she has a prosthetic eye because she tried to kill herself. I'm not sure if she tried to shoot herself or stab herself. But the eye is not hers, and that was just one of the attempts. There is such a sense of sadness surrounding her. She lost her husband; he died from cancer, suddenly. He loved her, and she believes she'll never find a love like that again. It's been about four or five years.

We were on the fourth floor, in the comfort suites (private rooms where patients and families can spend quality time at the end of life) – which means the loved one is likely to die very soon. I took our conversation back to her dad and asked her how she felt about his condition. *Honestly, I wondered how she could even be in the same room with him. I just couldn't wrap my mind around the things she was exposed to with this man. How could a father behave this way? I wondered when is enough, enough?* As our conversation continued she explained that she has a pretty good job, however, she is going through foreclosure. To complicate matters further, she doesn't have power of attorney for her father and he's not been able to speak.

Goodbye Daddy

Some Hope Is False

A doctor said there was some improvement in her father's condition and stated that putting a feeding tube in his stomach would extend his life. He didn't tell her how short the extension would be. When doctors don't consider the entire case and the impact of making "false hope" statements which lead to false hope decisions, it is maddening and inconsiderate in the long run. Why? Did the doctor not know that the family was in the grieving process? Did the doctor not know the impact of this stroke? The medical team educated the family and showed the images of this stroke. How pissed off my team became behind such false hope. Now he's on an inevitable journey. Life expectancy is measured in weeks to a month maybe. His condition is indeed an emotional rollercoaster for the family – the family, and this daughter who is on edge, ready for the trauma to be over. He will never be able to talk or walk and will always have respiratory problems, until he likely, aspirates and dies. What a way to live.

As the social worker, I told her about options for nursing home placement and finding a Medicare alternative to get him into a facility which would take him as they work through the process of paperwork and therapy. I added that after a few weeks, if there's no improvement, she needs to consider hospice and make final preparations.

She's ready to let him go now. She's ready. Either that or have a nervous breakdown and try and kill herself again. I told her that I couldn't fathom what she's going through. She was already in the pre-grieving stage; now she's in the confusion stage. I just wish the doctor had been forthcoming so that they would have known her father wasn't going to get better. It was a huge stroke and he won't come back from it. The likelihood of having another stroke is very high as well. I left the question with her, "How long are you going to let this go on and allow him to live this way?" "Would your dad want someone changing him, looking down on him and giving him 24-hour care?" "No, he wouldn't want to live like that," she said. So, there are regrets about the feeding tube now. It's there, and they can choose not to use it, that's after she sees if there is no improvement after a few weeks. Once in hospice, they can stop feeding through the tube, should she decide to go that route. I would have never put a feeding tube in a stroke patient who is that debilitated.

Her mom is bipolar. I wonder if she too inherited the condition? I can tell she was a daddy's girl. I could relate, because I was too. Though my father died of kidney failure, he died within days of being admitted to the hospital, so I didn't have to endure what she's going through with her father. Watching her dad go down, only able to move an arm, with confusing information, was traumatic. What I did go through was heartache, sadness, emptiness and anger after losing my father. I stayed like that for a long time because I felt like the only person who did love me was my father. In her case, it seems there is a love-hate relationship with her and her father. At least she knows he wouldn't want to live like that.

I gave her my business card and told her that we would get him placed. A few hours later we were able to place him in a nursing home. I feel she needs my help, and plan to be available for her, for her dad. Finally, I asked her to think of her children when she is thinking about her life – and preserving it or attempting to take it away again. She's a sad case and I'm worried she will try and take her life again. There are real, deep down embedded issues for which she will need professional assistance to help her cope. She's hiding behind a well-paid job; she's very professional and I would have never known about these issues had she not shared them with me.

Secrets from the past haunting adulthood have caused sadness, isolation and the lack of desire to be close to anyone, including her children. She loves them very much yet; the desire to kill herself is overwhelming 24 hours a day. With depression running through her family, she is reliving the cycle. She won't escape unless she gets the professional help she needs.

After her father passed, she did not return any of my phone calls. I prayed for her and her family. I don't know how I feel. I've learned to keep my feelings at bay. I had to learn not to let others' problems be my problems because when I did, I would develop a nervous condition.

Secrets often result in unresolved issues. Not addressing them only prolongs the pain and deepens generational issues. Opening up and treating problems, professionally, is a start to improving the quality of life for entire families.

Partying To Death

— ❦ —

"Turn up for what??? When I saw Luke lying in that bed, my heart dropped."

Too much was too much…

He was the father of a four-week-old baby girl, her four-year-old big sister, and had been celebrating his "Big 25" on the first of the month. Too much celebrating, he passed out from ingesting the alcohol and all the drugs. Heroin. Cocaine. Marijuana. Liquor. All together. It was all too much for his little-framed body.

Luke was found unconscious in the bathroom; no one knows how long. We know medically, it was for an extended period as there was swelling on the brain, and no "purposeful" life movement or existence.

How do you tell a mother and father that they will be burying their son? I tried keeping my emotions at bay as I thought about my own 24-year-old daughter and 10-month- old grandson; the thought of losing either of them would surely shatter my world. My tears dropped as I couldn't fight the emotions which overtook me.

Luke's mother sat in a catatonic state. She couldn't believe what was happening. She was numb as her husband held her in his arms. The girlfriend and mother of their two daughters cried and cried, she knew that this wasn't good. To see her grieving for herself and her children, and to hear that fingers were being pointed at her, as she was the one who found him in their home bathroom. The heart wrenching, blood-curdling cry she let out from her soul, was almost indescribable, a cry all too familiar to me. I felt her fears and the pain of not wanting to lose the support and love they'd shared for over five years. Her kids will be fatherless… How heartbreaking this is.

My team, the nurse practitioner, chaplain, intern chaplain and I were all present to comfort the family as a decision needed to be made. Over 35 family members crowded around as we explained that Luke's neurological report wasn't good and damage to his brain was irreversible…

Screeching, sobbing and outbursts filled the air. We sat in silence, giving the family time to allow the information to digest. No more words could be verbalized as the family stayed right there and could not process further.

Luke was gone on the fourth of the month.

"Be mindful of what you do and how you do it. Life, when young, seems eternal, and it's not. Your actions can hurt the people who love you the most, especially when you leave them behind."

The Last Script

— ✿ —

"Where's my doctor?"

"I'm sick!" My body is hurting and these nurses have said there's nothing else they can do. Can someone please call *my* doctor?" "Where is she?" "Is she in a meeting and can't be interrupted?" "Nurse, please get *my* doctor; I need medication for my pain! I need *my* doctor."

"Sir, I'm sorry, but the doctor is unavailable. The last script was written on the 24th."

He's not sure why the script can't be written by *his* doctor. We know, but we can't tell him. We will get the scripts written by another doctor.

"Please, lady. Please call *my* doctor; she knows everything about my condition. Trying to explain how I feel to someone else is exhausting and frustrating. And I don't want to do it."

She Was My Doctor Too

Before writing the last script, she was a wonderful, caring, kind-spirited woman who provided me with direction for a program which she created. She encouraged me to push myself when I failed my licensure exam. She told me, "Don't let a test define you as a person." She didn't use these words for herself when she was down. I'm hurting behind this tragedy. I didn't notice she was hurting.

I'm grateful for the good memories of her smiles. I can still picture our conversations as she clicked the end of her ballpoint pen as she spoke to me. I can still hear her quick steps going "clickety-clack" as she graced the stairwells and hallways visiting her patients. I remember the constant spills during morning rounds as her coffee met her white lab jacket. What a wonderful person she was! I do miss her. A fierce leader, she was exceptional to work with, and the patients and families felt the same way.

I miss my doctor!

We often take for granted that we will see each other, especially those we work with, the next day. When that doesn't happen, our expectations go unmet; our schedules are interrupted and depending on the circumstances; our lives may never be the same.

Loss happens and it's especially unique in the medical community as it's sometimes impossible or inappropriate to discuss with patients what has happened. When you think of loved ones and cherished friends,
Speak Up Before It's Too Late!

Breaking Point

— ❀ —

"Why suicide? I'll never understand."

It was premeditated, I know it was. To me, suicide is always pre-mediated. It starts with a thought, and it is acted upon. At low points, the depression is too deep, but the thoughts are planted. At higher points, the thoughts and plans are laid out. And then at some point, the action is taken.

It was devastating. In my mind, I just suppressed it and told myself she had a heart attack. I don't talk about it and have felt uncomfortable whenever someone else mentions her. She kept things very professional with me. I didn't even know her favorite color. I just don't understand how she was sustaining and saving people every day, yet she was in such a dark place in her life. I didn't know she was in a dark place. I would have never expected her to do that, never.

Her desk was always sloppy. Each week I would go in and wipe off her desk before I left for the weekend. I don't know why I just did it, it seemed like the right thing to do, I like to spoil my crew. This particular Friday her desk was cleaned off. I didn't think anything of it and just went about my business and left for the evening. I got a call Saturday from my team, letting me know she had died. It devastated me. I cried. My grief was compounded with a lot of emotion, as I had just lost my aunt, and it was right around Father's Day. I got overwhelmed. I just dealt with it. I cried all day Saturday, off and on. The thought that she was gone was just overwhelming.

She was a very humble lady. She was thoughtful, compassionate and gave excellent care. I think I'm also angry that she left her family behind, and of course, that she left us behind. I do have some guilt since I saw her that Thursday, she wasn't at work Friday and Saturday she took her own life. I gasped and cried from the pit of my stomach and it triggered so many thoughts inside.

Years Ago My Friend Lee Committed Suicide

I was blamed for it, his suicide that is. His family thought I was his girlfriend and that he took his life out of rejection. However, I wasn't. I had a boyfriend. Lee wanted to date me, but I was a full-time student and doing an internship at the time.

I shared with him that I didn't want to lose focus with what I was doing. In actuality, he was not my type. Growing up as the only girl, I saw myself as a tomboy, but dainty in appearance. I was rough with verbiage, but never intentionally hurt people with outward rejection.

He came to my house one Friday morning, wanting to talk, and I invited him in. He sat on the couch and accused me of saying, "The sight of him makes me sick," as he heard from a mutual friend. I told him that wasn't true. I didn't say that. If memory serves me, he started apologizing to me and said he would make it right. I wondered what he meant by "making it right," but I didn't ask. He seemed stoic, with a flat affect and kept saying, "I'm going to make this right." He was about 6'2" and frail. When he grabbed both of my hands in one of his large hands, I felt a certain way, and I snatched my hands out from under his. It was hot. He kept one hand in his pocket. He was jittery and acting weird. I was wondering why he was wearing the jacket and why he continued to keep that one hand in the pocket. He kept saying "I want to make this right. Tell your mom I'm sorry for calling her house and cussing at her, looking for you." I just knew it was time for him to go. I told him I had to leave for work. As he was walking out my front door, I couldn't see his reflection in the mirror which was actually there.

The look on his face wasn't right when I looked directly at him. It was strange. After he left, I didn't think anything else of it and went to my internship.

When I got home, my mother called and said, "Lee started calling about one o'clock, checking to see if you were home. He kept calling and I kept telling him no, and to stop calling. Finally, I told him you had a boyfriend and hung up." I asked my mother why she would tell him that. It wasn't the time or place for her to say that to him. She didn't have a response. That's just how she is; blunt, and not caring if she hurts your feelings. She didn't care about his feelings; she just wanted him to stop calling her house looking for me.

About nine that same night, someone knocked on the door. It was Raymond, Lee's best friend. He said, "Lee is gone." I said, "What do you mean he's gone?" He said, "Bitch, Lee's gone!" He gestured his hand with a gun to his head. I cried out and fell out. My boyfriend came running downstairs, asking what was going on. In between sobbing and being in disbelief, I told him Lee killed himself. He too was shocked.

Raymond told me to come down the street, to Lee's house then he left. After I gathered myself from screaming, my mother, boyfriend and I got into the car and went to Lee's house. The yard and house were full of people. I remember walking in. Everyone was crying, and everyone knew who I was for some reason, yet I didn't know who most of them were.

I saw a familiar face, his grandfather, and gave him a hug, then asked what happened. He said, "I'm glad you're okay. It would have been a murder-suicide. He went to your house to kill you first. When he called and you weren't home, he went upstairs to his bedroom and killed himself." His grandparents had been downstairs and heard the pop. When they opened the door, the room was a complete mess. Along with his lifeless body, they found the gun he used to kill himself and also a machete.

I immediately wondered if my mother's conversation with him had pushed him over the edge. I told his grandfather that I didn't know he was in that state of mind, not getting the seriousness of where he was from our earlier conversation. His grandfather said he had been sick in the head for a long time. Evidently, he had been going into rages on his job and doing other odd things, like punching holes in the walls at home and in public places. When I heard that, I knew it was some type of mental illness and that I wasn't the cause of his suicide.

During the time I was in the house, his sister called my name and walked up saying, "Lee said it's not your fault. Lee said it was not her fault. He was going to take your life with his. I want everyone to hear this! It's not Beverly's fault!" His mother walked up behind me saying, "You bitch, you took my son from me. You bitch. You bitch, you took my son. You're the second bitch who took my sons' life." I told her I didn't. She repeated her accusations. I began walking out of the house, hyperventilating. It hurt. It cut like a bunch of knives. I was also confused. I didn't know, at the time what she meant. Later I learned Lee's brother had committed suicide as well. At the moment, she was in my face. I was hurt, angry and she was cussing me out because she was hurt and angry. Reflecting, if I were in my right frame of mind, I would have sealed her mouth with my fist with that word I so hate... bitch.

His grandfather told me to go home. I did.

I went to my college counselor the next day, that Monday, after he killed himself, telling her I wanted to withdraw from school. She convinced me to stay in school. I only had one month left before graduation with my Bachelor's Degree. She got me the help I needed and I did graduate, on time.

At the wake, his mother told me not to cry for her son. She whispered, "Get your face together, don't be up there crying. I know now, it's not your fault." Her statement gave me some type of comfort, yet my friend was gone. When I saw him lying in the casket, he looked good. You couldn't see his cock eye or his buck teeth. But it wasn't just his appearance that was different. Depression and darkness ran in his family. No more living in turmoil, captured by schizophrenia, coupled by auditory hallucinations. In the casket, finally, he was at peace.

The thought of what happened was still bothering me. I remember coming onto my front porch pulling my hair, screaming and crying, escaping from the house, feeling like I heard Lee's voice speaking to me, haunting me; but his words were always, "I'm sorry." A pastor's wife was outside and saw me. I yelled, "I'm tired of being blamed for this shit! I can't take it anymore!" She immediately started praying for me. That Sunday I went to church. The pastor looked at me through my tears and said, "It's not your fault." I knew right then God was speaking to me through him, assuring me it wasn't my fault for Lee's suicide and that it was okay to let it go. That day my healing began. I'm still a member of that church, 15 years later.

My church experience has taught me so much about faith, life, illness and coping with loss. When my supervisor committed suicide many years later, I didn't feel it was my fault, though it was difficult to deal with. Years and perspective helped. However, I certainly wish she had felt comfortable enough to allow me in to help her through the dark time, instead of taking her life.

Thinking about Lee and my supervisor brings up certain feelings. It's alright to feel. It's sad when you suppress everything and don't allow yourself to feel. Then when you do allow yourself to feel, it won't come out because it's been pushed back for so long. Everyone copes with death/suicide differently. The important thing is to cope and not to give up or give into darkness. I just keep looking at her name. I still see stars when I look at her name. When I look at Lee's name, I still see darkness. I wonder if there is anything I could have done differently with either one.

Suicide is something I will never understand. I'll never understand the reason behind the why and the why behind the reason.

If you don't open the door and allow people to support you, you end up committing suicide, especially when you are overwhelmed. People think they don't have a way out, but we do.

Tears for Daddy

— ❧ —

"I was disturbed because I saw myself in her, crying for her father. I saw her and me crying, though I wasn't crying on the outside."

On the last Friday in July, the daughter was breaking down crying, grieving for the only father she had known, lay dying. This man, who had married her mother when she was three years old, only had herself with her two babies. He had a limited support system. Her mother had divorced him years ago and left them both to fend for themselves.

She kept saying how much he loved her sons and her. The only person who I believe loved her was her dad. Her mother did not console her; she looked at her daughter with virtually no feeling as she continued to grieve. "I'm good, I'm good," is all she could manage to say as she attempted to process what we had just told her about her dad's health and short life expectancy. It had been a lot for her to take in, a lot for which she was not ready.

While doing my rounds Monday morning, I walked into Damon's room to check on him around 9:30. Though he was still breathing, I "saw" a dead corpse. He had a pooling of tears in his eyes. No words were spoken. I just said, in my spirit, *Goodbye.* He died at 11:50 am. They held his body until 4 pm in the ICU, waiting for the family. Nobody showed. He died the way he lived. Alone and rejected.

When people don't show it's usually because they are at work, they don't want to, or they just can't bear to put any more grief into their bags. They are just done. When I found out the daughter didn't show it saddened me just a bit. I know it was hard for her. She had nothing left.

I followed up and reiterated the offer to get support for her and her 11-year-old, asking had she made the call. She hadn't and didn't intend to.

Framing things a certain way, offering support and suggesting resources is a large part of what I do. I can lead someone to water, but I can't make them drink...

What Hospice Is And Isn't

—— ❦ ——

Often people get confused about Hospice Care, thinking hospice is a place people go to die, and it is not. Hospice is a specialized type of care for those facing life-limiting illnesses, taking a holistic approach, considering the mind, body and spirit. Another way to say that is treating the emotional, physical, social and spiritual needs of the patient. Normally, two doctors have to agree that the patient is hospice eligible, with a terminal diagnosis of six months or less to live. Once hospice is ordered, an interdisciplinary team of professionals consisting of the medical doctor, the nurse, the social worker, the home health aide and the chaplain work together to care for patient needs. Each has their respective duties to serve the patient, with the doctor overseeing the entire case.

All orders go through the doctor, including the plan of care and managing pain medication dosages. The nurse serves as the liaison between the doctor and others and leads the case. The home health aide bathes and cleans the patient while keeping them as comfortable as possible. Many conversations occur between the aide and the patient because of the nature of their relationship, the physical contact, and the time spent with the patient.

The social worker attends to the patient as well as to the patients' family, including advance care planning, educating the family about the disease, the hospice plan and journey, and supports their adjusting to the process and progress during hospice and preparing for finality, after hospice. This often includes end of life planning and offering a supportive ear where family members may express any issues or concerns so that the loved one can have a peaceful transition. This can include grief support and addressing resource needs like food, bills, last wishes and the like.

The chaplain offers a supportive presence, offering prayer and guidance, as well as dealing with any fears or spiritual distress a patient may have.

About Hospice:

- Can be rendered in a home setting, nursing home, inpatient hospital setting for short-term or symptom management, or in an assisted living setting;

- Is a specialized type of care for those facing a life-limiting illness, usually six months or less, some do live longer;
- Specialty services include, but are not limited to massage, music, and pet therapy;
- Is covered 100% under Medicare;
- Medications related to the diagnosis including an emergency comfort pack, are covered by Medicare;
- The emergency comfort pack includes agitation, nausea, and diarrhea medications; suppositories for fevers and constipation; as well as medication for pain and respiratory distress – usually morphine;
- Medicare covered hygiene supplies include: a disposable bed pad (Chux), adult diapers, powders, body creams and ointments for wounds/sores, razors, shaving creams, etc. Each of these items is covered though some hospice providers will not supply them;
- Medical equipment includes a hospital bed, an over-the-bed table, an oxygen concentrator with tanks, a bedside commode, a wheelchair, and a broader chair (a padded, reclining chair which allows the patient to be comfortable when not in the bed).

Dispelling Myths of Hospice

- No, hospice is not a place;
- Being in hospice does not mean giving up hope;
- Being assigned to hospice offers comfort, support and presence when medical options have been exhausted. It does not mean "nothing else" can be done.
- Is not about "just dying" or "giving up control," it is about choices and how the patient desires their last days to be lived out.
- Hospice is not only for people 65 years and older, on Medicare - even five-year-olds with a terminal diagnosis can receive hospice care.
- The primary care doctor can be kept, through the end of life, if the patient and doctor agree to do so. This often helps the patient in feeling more comfortable, because of established rapport;
- Hospice is not only for the patient, but the entire family also goes on hospice and receives treatment/care; even family pets that have close relationships with the patient tend to know when the end is near.

Don't let myths about hospice keep you or your loved ones from utilizing the services. Hospice is an entitlement.
It's free and anyone who needs it should use it.

Palliative Care

—— ✿ ——

"The primary aim of palliative care is to give quality comfort by providing assistance to the patient and treating symptoms associated with a chronic illness."

Palliative, Pronounced (Pal-lee-uh-tiv)

Unlike hospice care, which is given after diagnosis, palliative care may begin at the point of diagnosis or treatment and does not only deal with illnesses which inevitably lead to death. For example, kidney failure is a primary example of a non-curable disease which may be managed through dialysis while the patient is waiting for a kidney transplant. In the event a kidney transplant is not an option, dialysis treatment can continue over the course of years until other organs begin to fail or the patient no longer wants dialysis.

Palliative Care offers supportive services where a team of professionals work to alleviate the patient's symptoms. The team is not there to "cure" but to "manage" symptoms and improve the quality of life.

Palliative Care Overview

- Specialized medical care for people with serious illness;
- Focuses on providing relief from the symptoms and stress of serious illness;
- Goal is to improve quality of life for both the patient and the family;
- Is a multidiscipline approach, incorporating a palliative care medical doctor, nurse practitioner, social worker and chaplain;
- Appropriate at any age and any stage in a serious illness, whether that illness is curable, chronic, or life-threatening;
- Can be provided at a hospital, a nursing home, an assisted-living facility, or at home;
- Many private insurance companies and health maintenance organizations (HMOs) offer palliative care as a benefit. Medicare plan (Part B) may offer it, varying by state.

Medical Considerations

— ❧ —

"Medical terms can be confusing."

DNR, DNI and Intubation

- Do Not Resuscitate (**DNR**) is a medical order written by a doctor instructing health care providers not to perform cardiopulmonary resuscitation (CPR) if a patient's breathing stops or if the heart stops beating.
- The DNR goes in hand with the (**DNI**) Do Not Intubate, instructing health care providers not to perform intubation when a patient is having trouble breathing before the heart stops.
- **Intubation** is when a medical professional inserts a flexible plastic tube through the nose or mouth into the trachea, or windpipe, to help with breathing. The tube is usually connected to a machine called a ventilator which pushes oxygen into the patient's lungs.

Power of Attorney/Advanced Medical Directive

- Power of Attorney (**POA**) is a written document giving someone permission to represent or act on another's behalf. It can be business, medical or personal. The POA authorizes the other person to act as the principal, grantor or donor.
- The **Advanced Medical Directive** document is intended to honor the patient's medical wishes.

Caregiver Stress

Caregiver stress is the emotional and physical strain of caregiving. It can manifest in many forms, including feelings of frustration and anger.

Example: Lamont has been taking care of his elderly mother for 10 years, who is stricken with Alzheimer's disease. He voices with anger his frustrations related to not having enough. He gets tearful that he doesn't get a break; he's tied to the home because he doesn't have help caring for his mother, leaving to chance going to the grocery store. He's feeling confined, with limited interaction with family and friends. He doesn't have social outlets to express himself… Lamont is exhibiting all the signs of caregiver stress.

Dealing with Difficult Personalities

Dealing with difficult people and their personalities during serious or terminal illness takes patience and reasoning. As a family member or professional, it's important to see that they are going through emotional and mental turmoil and that the result can be quite overwhelming. Naturally difficult people tend to lash out in an abrasive, often verbally abusive manner. You must ask yourself if is it intentional, if they are just rude, or if this is a coping mechanism. Once you adjust your thinking, make some choices to deal with them.

- Keep calm, don't feed into their feelings.
- Don't take what they are saying personally.
- Do what you can to de-escalate the situation.
- Listen to what they are saying and acknowledge them and their feelings.
- Be genuine. Show concern.
- Ask for mutual respect and come to a mutually agreeable compromise when appropriate.
- Seek help in volatile situations.

The Grief Process

Grief starts when the reality of the loss becomes real. Anxiety sets in; trying to channel this energy becomes overwhelming to most people. There are five stages of grief:

1. Denial: Disbelief that this is actually happening and eventually, death is going to occur.
2. Anger: You're angry at the person for the anticipated inevitable. Anger has no limits. During this stage, acknowledge what you are feeling. It's always good to journal during such a delicate time to express yourself.
3. Bargaining: Trying to ask a higher power for more time. Negotiating as well as exploring the "what ifs…"
4. Acceptance: You have decided what will happen, will happen and the person will transition.
5. Depression (Misery): You feel withdrawn, with intense, prolonged sadness.

When grieving, own your feelings, talk about what is hurting you regarding the anticipated demise of your loved one. During any of these stages, give permission to the person to die. Honor the person and your memories.

A Note From The Publisher

—— ❦ ——

Mission Possible Press...
Creating Legacies through Absolute Good Works

As a publisher, I have the opportunity to transform hopeful writers into successful authors. This brings me great pleasure because I believe everyone has wisdom to share and valuable stories to tell.

Being a caring person while facing some of the most difficult circumstances daily takes strength, courage and character. Sharing deep pain while being open and optimistic takes a calling, one I know Beverly Dotson is answering. Beverly shows us all how to be our best selves during the most difficult times.

Thanks to Beverly Dotson, we are continuing to make the *Mission Possible-creating legacies, inspiring and building up- especially for families.*

I am honored and pleased to present this book, *Goodbye Daddy, Speak Up Before It's Too Late,* as part of our Extraordinary Living Series.

In the Spirit of Communication,
Jo Lena Johnson, Founder and Publisher

Mission Possible Press, a division of Absolute Good
AbsoluteGoodbooks.com
MissionPossiblePress.com

About The Author

—— ❧ ——

Beverly Dotson is a dedicated MSW who has been working, educating and providing resources to underserved populations via hospice, home health, mentoring, palliative care and community outreach. A graduate of the University of Missouri with a Masters Certificate in Non-profit Management in Leadership, she holds a Master's degree from the St. Louis University School of Social Work, and is a graduate of Fontbonne University, with double minors in Psychology and Sociology.

Beverly currently works at Christian Hospital as the Palliative Care Social Worker and continues to serve as a hospice social worker, which she has done for over 12 years. Beverly works with people of diverse backgrounds, tackling barriers to overcome challenges in health care while dispelling common myths in Urban communities which often keep families from making informed choices and utilizing available services. An active volunteer, she works with *The Empowerment*

Network as the Secretary, serving men who are stricken and survivors of prostate cancer. Beverly also is a co-host of the *Healthy Focus Radio Show*, a weekly show airing in the St. Louis metropolitan area, where she calls home. Beverly is the proud mother of a 25-year-old daughter and one-year-old grandson.

Acknowledgements

— ✿ —

To my beautiful and dedicated daughter, Desiray, *Reach until you can't reach anymore and never let anyone take you off your course. If they aren't adding to the substance of your being, they don't deserve you.*

To my mother, brothers and family, thanks for all the love and support you've given me throughout the years.

Thanks, Katina Beane and Katrina Agnew, my mentors and friends, for always believing in me, pushing me, inspiring me and for your relentless work ethic, and passion. Your presence and words remind me to never give up.

Thanks to my publisher and literary coach, Ms. Jo Lena Johnson for believing in me; saying, "I have a book inside me." Without your push, motivation and kindred spirit, I would probably still be thinking, wondering if I could actually do this. I truly thank Mr. and Mrs. Kenric Williams for initiating Jo Lena's and my divine connection.

Thank you to my friends/colleagues near and far for all the support, you've given; from kind words and gestures to encouraging me. Because of the nature of our work, I won't name you individually; however, you are cherished and special to me. This includes my social worker colleagues for cheerleading me through endless support and gatherings; and you, my doctors: Primary Care Physicians, Specialists, Hospice, Palliative Care, Medical Students, Nurse Techs, Chaplains, and Nurse Practitioners.

To the families who play a major role in this book, these are your stories and I am sharing them with your permission. Words of thank you aren't enough, but yet, Thank you!!!

The highest accolades go to My GOD; thank you for what you have allowed these eyes to see and live through; and thank you for trusting me to serve you, my colleagues, my patients and their families. Thank you, LORD.